JENNIFER ROMAN

5 Minute Workouts

Quick Exercises to Help Maximize Fat Loss And Increase Energy

This book was professionally typeset on Reedsy.
Find out more at reedsy.com

Contents

1

Introduction

This book is to serve as a mini guide to some quick, energy boosting, fat burning workouts that you can do in about 5 minutes.

I decided to put this handbook together from my love of fitness and exercise. I've been dedicated to fitness for the past 15 years and use this as a tool to start my days, to help clear my mind, to de-stress, etc. Whatever the situation, I find that taking a few minutes out of your day to do one, some, or even all of these exercises can have such a positive impact on not just your physical health, but your mental and emotional health as well.

Before you start any kind of program or routine, it's helpful to give yourself a realistic goal. You should decide what it is you're trying to obtain. Is it fat loss? Is it to boost metabolism? Gain muscle? And remember, it will not happen overnight. It's important to not get discouraged if you don't see results within a few days of working out. If you stick to it, before you know it, your clothes will start fitting differently, you'll eventually start to see results...but only if you stick with it. Don't be ruled by the scale either. A scale can be useful if your goal is strictly to drop pounds…but weigh yourself on a schedule, not every day. Shoot for weekly, or even monthly. Because scales can also be the one tool that discourages many people. Sometimes, as you gain muscle and drop fat, you'll become leaner, your clothes will fit you looser, but the scale may not have changed – or it could even go up, as muscle does weigh more than fat.

It's also important for you to carve out the time that works best for you in your day. Some people prefer working out in the morning, as it gives them a boost of energy to help push them through their days. Some prefer the evenings to unwind after a stressful day at work or with the kids. Some people like to break their days up with a quick workout in the afternoon. And some people will simply get the workout in whenever their schedule allows. It doesn't matter. It all depends on what works for you.

2

Getting Started

Before getting started make sure that you have an adequate amount of water. Also make sure you have enough space, whether it be at a gym, at your home, outside, etc. Make sure that you won't accidentally bang into something to prevent a possible injury. A towel is something you should have on hand too. Although these exercises can be done in 5 minutes, you can work up a sweat, and you can also combine them to create a longer workout. A good pair of sneakers or tennis shoes are recommended to avoid slipping or sliding on any particular surface. Some exercises can be performed barefoot, but just be careful considering that with all of them. Injuries can occur.

You can grab some dumbbells - be sure to not go too heavy. You can risk injury if you're using weights that are too heavy. If you don't have weights, you can always improvise with things around the house. Water bottles, food cans, even packets of rice or beans can replace dumbbells. Resistance bands are another popular way to add some strength training to your workouts. This is all totally dependent on your goals and your fitness level.

3

Workouts

L et's get into the workouts. Keep in mind, you can do any of these for longer than 5 minutes, should you so choose.You can combine several of these together for a longer workout too.

<u>BODYWEIGHT CIRCUIT -</u> A Bodyweight Circuit will target multiple muscle groups, burn fat, and enhance your overall fitness. With this, you'd come up with 5 exercises. Do each one for the full minute, and immediately switch to the next. You can do things like Deep Squats, Lunges, Pushups, Planks, Mountain Climbers, Wall Sit, High Knees, Seated Leg Tucks.

Deep Squats - Start with feet shoulder width apart, and descend until your hips are below the height of your knees. Explode up to starting position, and repeat. You can incorporate weight (a dumbbell, barbell, medicine ball, etc) if you want to add resistance.

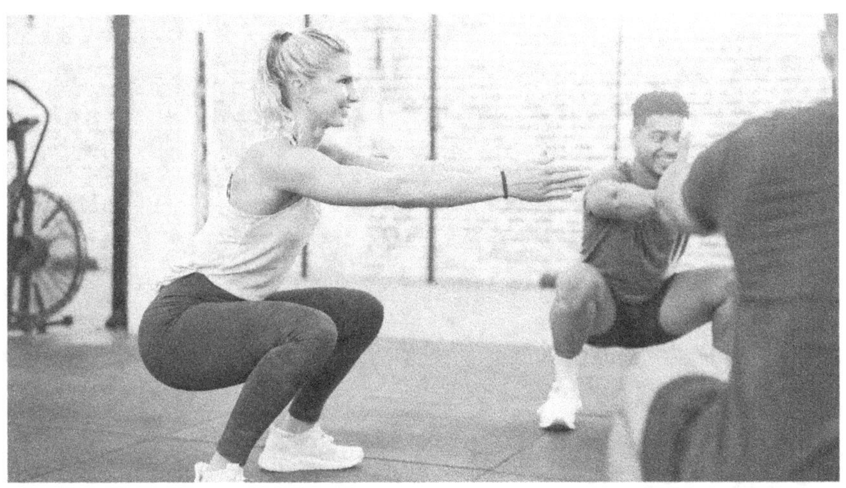

Lunges – These can be forward lunges or reverse lunges. Forward Lunges, you would step forward with one foot and lower your hips so that both your front leg and back leg are bent at an approximate 90 degree angle. Return to starting position then repeat with the other foot. You can add dumbbells (or water bottles) for some added resistance.

Reverse Lunges are similar to Forward Lunges, except instead of stepping forward, you would take a large step back and do the same thing as the Forward Lunge. Again, weights can be incorporated, should you choose to add some resistance. Make sure to keep your core tight and engaged during the exercise.

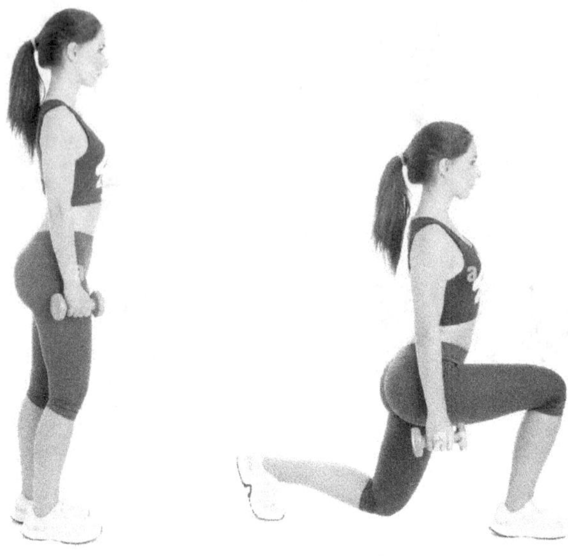

Pushups - Start in a prone position with your hands, palms down, under your shoulders. The balls of your feet should be on the ground, your back should be straight, core tight. Push your body up, straighten your arms, and then lower it down again by bending your elbows.There are many variations to this exercise. Instead of being on the balls of your feet, you can be on your knees as a lesser degree of difficulty. You can do standing push ups, using a wall to push off from. You can also change your hand position to target your muscles from different angles.

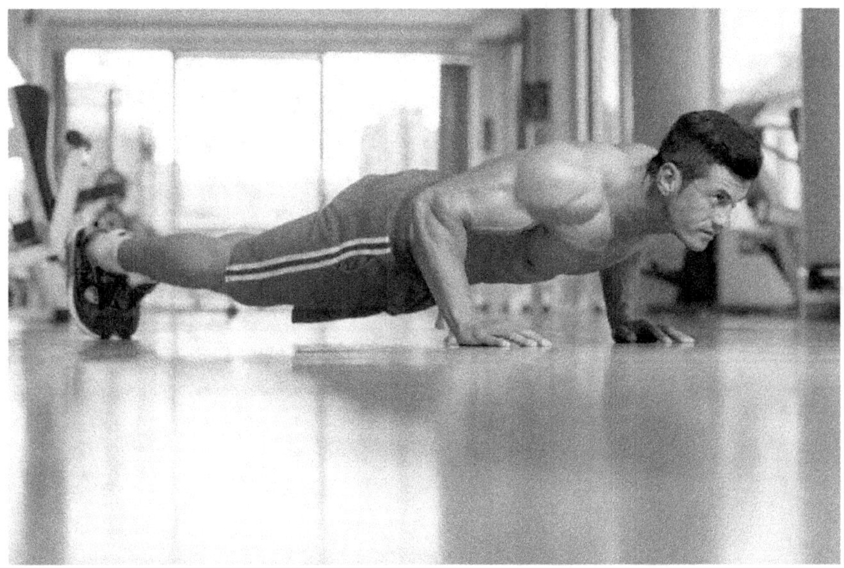

Planks - In this exercise, you hold your body straight and parallel to the floor. You should be on your toes, and your hands palms down. Or you can be on your elbows. This exercise is meant to engage and strengthen your core. Hold this position for as long as you can without compromising your form.

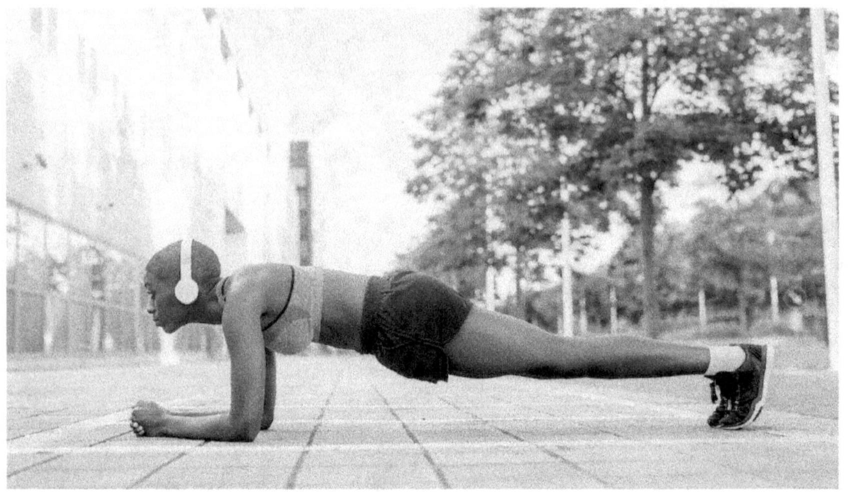

Mountain Climbers - Mountain Climbers should be performed starting in a plank position (described above). You would begin by bringing one knee up towards your chest, then back out, alternating with the other knee to your chest. As you gain speed, it should almost simulate running against the floor.

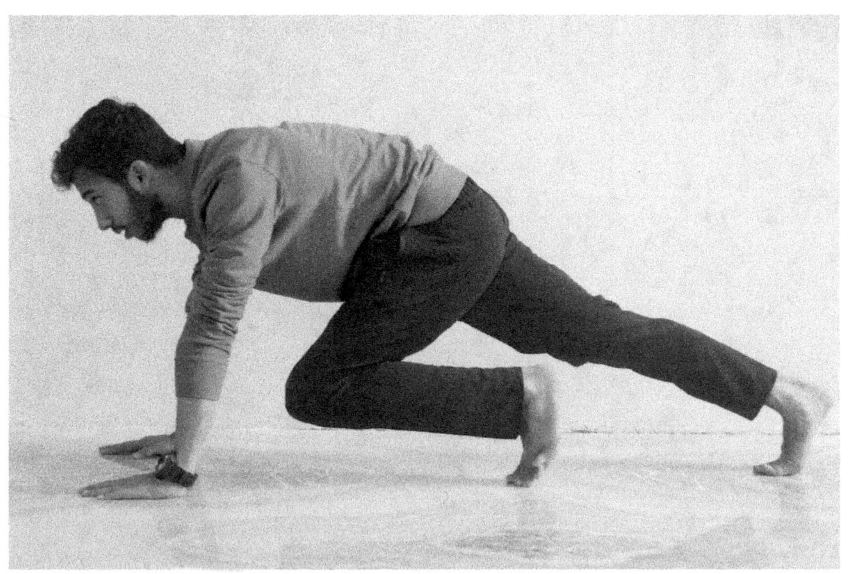

Wall Sit - Wall Sits are difficult and many people start struggling maintaining proper form a minute into doing them. So don't be discouraged. Stand with feet shoulder width apart and about 1.5 to 2 feet away from the wall. Keeping your core tight and engaged, slide your back down the wall until your legs are bent at a 90 degree angle, in a sitting position. Someone should be able to come over and place something on your lap without it falling or sliding off. Hold this position for 1 minute.

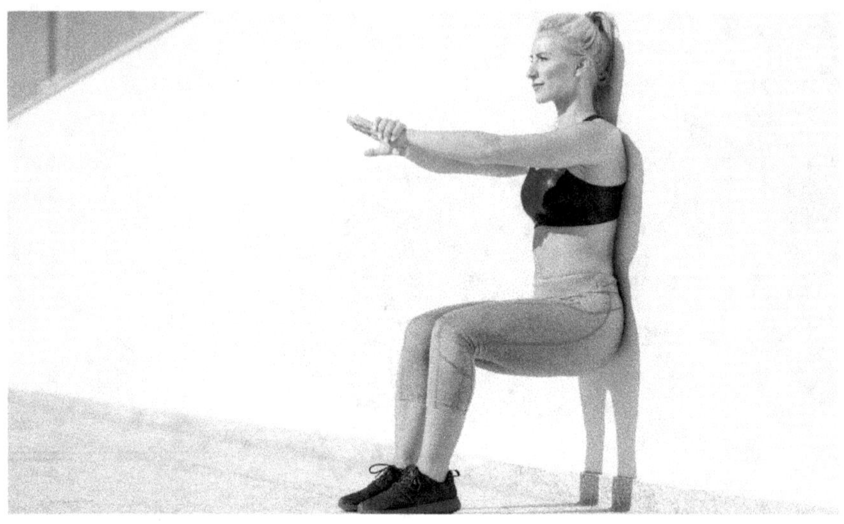

High Knees - High Knees are similar to a march, or running in place, but exaggerated because you're bringing your knees up towards your chest. You can start slow at first until you get the correct movement down, then increase the pace. This is a great exercise to get your blood flowing.

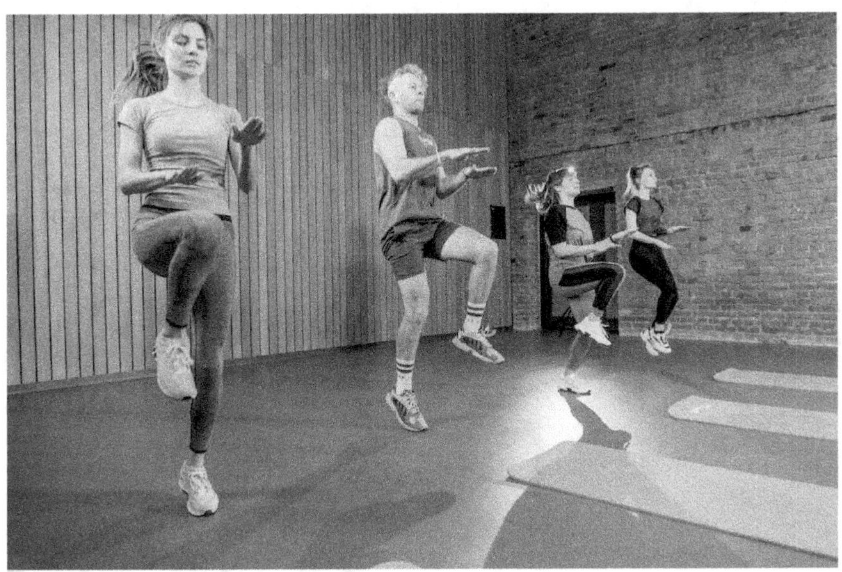

Seated Leg Tucks - Sit on the floor (or a mat) with your hands, palms down, at your sides. Your elbows should be slightly bent. Your legs are out straight, raised in the air. Tuck your knees towards you, bringing them to your chest. Pause, then return to the starting position. For this exercise, do not forget to breathe. It sounds silly, but people tend to hold their breath for this exercise. As you get more comfortable, you can pick your hands up and place them behind your head for a more advanced workout.

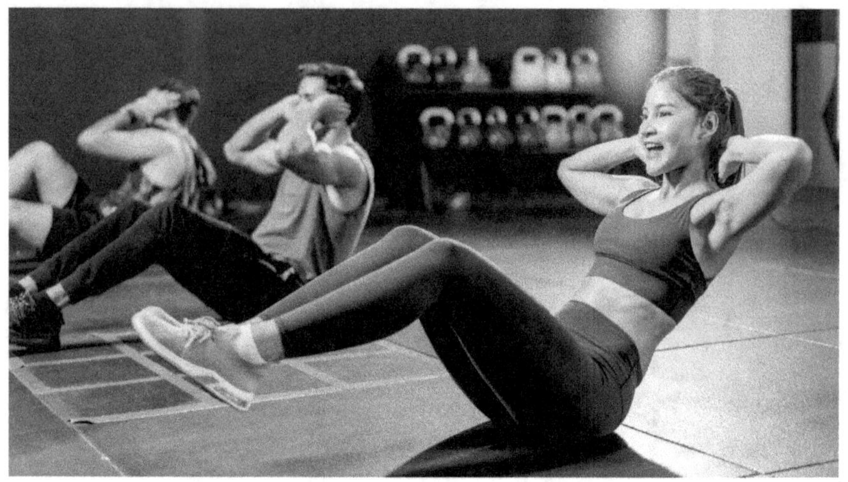

HIIT - HIIT stands for High Intensity Interval Training. It consists of short bursts of high intensity exercise, followed by a short rest, or low intensity exercise. You can do this in increments of 45 seconds of high intensity, followed by 15 seconds of low intensity.

You can do 5 minutes of any of the exercises below. If you want a longer workout, you can combine them for whatever length of time you're comfortable with. HIIT is very intense to make sure to take a break if you feel dizzy, nauseous, or lightheaded. HIIT is known to boost metabolism and maximize calorie burning.

Some examples of HIIT are:

Jumping Jacks. Do jumping jacks for 45 seconds as fast as you can. Followed by 15 seconds of toe taps. Repeat this for 5 minutes.

Burpees. Burpees are everyone's favorite (sarcasm). Burpees are done by standing upright, drop to the ground and do a pushup, pull your feet into your chest, hop up with a jump. Repeat. These are brutal, but so worth it. You can do them for 45 seconds, and give yourself a 15 second breather walking in place. Repeat this for 5 minutes.

Jumping Rope. Self explanatory. Jump rope as intensely as you can, without hurting yourself, for 45 seconds, then slow it down and do bodyweight squats for 15 seconds. Repeat this for 5 minutes.

Sprinting. You can sprint in place if you're indoors, 45 seconds running in place as fast as you can, then slowing it down to a march for 15 seconds. Repeat for 5 minutes. If you're outside you can give yourself a specific distance. Say, sprint to the end of your block, then walk back, then repeat.

TABATA – Tabata workouts are similar to HIIT as it is also done using intervals, but Tabata follows a specific timed interval structure. It's meant to maximize fat burning. Tabata is done in 20 seconds of high intense exercise, followed by 10 seconds of rest, immediately moving back into the 20 seconds of high intense exercise. This can be any exercise, as long as you do it with max intensity, followed by 10 seconds of rest.

Some suggestions for Tabata exercises are:

Squat Jumps – Bodyweight squats would be best to start out with, but as you gain experience and your fitness level increases, you can begin to incorporate some light weights. Start standing feet shoulder width apart, with your weight on your heels. Bend your knees into a squat and drive up through your heels to a jump. Repeat this for 5 minutes.

Pushups – Beginning in a prone position, hands palm facing down under your chest, core tight. Legs out straight, on the balls of your feet. Lift your body as you straighten your arms, then bend your elbows to lower your chest back down to the floor, getting as close to the floor as you can, without touching it. Do as many as you can for 20 seconds. Followed by 10 seconds of rest. Repeat that for 5 minutes.

Mountain Climbers – In plank position, alternate bringing your knees to your chest. For 20 seconds, then rest for 10. Repeat for 5 minutes.

Speed Skaters – Start knees slightly bent, feet should be wider than your hips. Cross right leg behind the left, bending your left knee, then drive off your left foot to hop to the right, landing on your right foot, letting your left leg cross behind the right. Keep lateral hopping for 20 seconds, rest for 10. Repeat for 5 minutes.

You can switch and combine any of the HIIT and Tabata exercises cross functionally.

JUMP ROPE – Jumping Rope is a fantastic cardio exercise. You can create a routine of your own by alternating between the way you jump, i.e. regular jumps, high knees, double unders, etc. Jumping Rope is great for improving your cardiovascular health and endurance.

YOGA – Yoga is great to improve flexibility, strength, and balance. You can do just a few moves each day and incorporate more as you become familiar with the many different yoga poses. Poses like Warrior Sequences and Sun Salutations are probably your best poses to start with. Remember to focus on controlled movements and deep breathing.

There are plenty of other exercises you can do if you're looking to burn fat, speed up your metabolism and increase your energy. It's important to mix things up. A key to keeping your metabolism burning optimally is to not let yourself get stuck in the same routine for too long. You want to fool your metabolism a little bit.

In between these workouts listed, you could do things like cycling, swimming, jogging, hitting the weights for some strength training. Building muscle will help you burn fat better as well. Remember to combine any exercise with a balanced diet for optimal fat burning results. If you have underlying health conditions, always make sure to consult with a healthcare provider or fitness professional before starting any new routine.

4

Maintaining Energy Levels

Tips to help you maximize and sustain your energy levels throughout your day are:

- Stay Hydrated. Dehydration can lead to fatigue. Make sure to drink an adequate amount of water throughout your day, whether exercising or not. Carry a water bottle with you to make sure you're getting enough water.
- Balanced Diet. Eat a well-balanced diet with a mix of carbohydrates, proteins, and healthy fats. Include whole grains, lean proteins, fruits, vegetables, and nuts in your meals to provide a steady source of energy.
- Regular meals. Instead of large meals, infrequently throughout your day, try eating smaller meals, more frequently, to maintain stable blood sugar levels. This helps prevent energy crashes.
- Limit your sugar and refined carbs. While carbohydrates are important, choose complex carbs over refined ones. Limit your intake of sugary snacks and drinks, as they can

cause rapid energy spikes - followed by hard crashes.

- Prioritize Sleep. Aim for 7-9 hours of quality sleep per night. Lack of sleep can significantly impact energy levels. Establish a consistent sleep routine and create a comfortable sleep environment.
- Exercise regularly. Engage in regular physical activity. Exercise improves circulation, boosts mood, and increases energy levels. Aim for at least 150 minutes of exercise per week. You can gauge your intensity level.
- Manage stress levels. Chronic stress can lead to fatigue. Practice stress management techniques such as deep breathing, meditation, or yoga to keep stress level in check.
- Power naps. A short nap, around 20-30 minutes, can help refresh your mind and boost alertness. Avoid napping for too long, as it may interfere with nighttime sleep.
- Limit caffeine intake. While caffeine can provide a temporary energy boost, excessive intake can lead to crashes and disrupt sleep. Consume caffeine in moderation and avoid it in the late afternoon and evening.
- Sunlight exposure. Spend some time outdoors to get some natural sunlight. Sunlight helps regulate your circadian rhythm and can improve your mood and energy levels.
- Socialize and take breaks. Taking short breaks and spending time with friends or colleagues can provide a mental energy boost. Social interactions can be invigorating.
- Set realistic goals. Break down your tasks into manageable goals. Achieving small victories can boost your confidence and motivation, leading to sustained energy.

Remember that every individual's energy needs vary, and it's essential to listen to your body. If you consistently struggle with low energy levels, it's advisable to consult with a healthcare professional to rule out any underlying health issues.

5

Sticking to Your Workout Goals

S ticking to workout goals can be challenging, but with the right mindset and strategies, you can increase your chances of success. Here are some tips to help you stay committed to your workout routine:

- Set realistic goals. Define clear, achievable and realistic fitness goals. Break down larger goals into smaller, manageable milestones. This makes the journey more attainable and less overwhelming.
- Create a schedule. Plan your workouts in advance and incorporate them into your weekly schedule. Treat them as non-negotiable appointments. Consistency is key to building a habit.
- Find activities you enjoy. Choose workouts or physical activities that you genuinely enjoy. Whether it's running, dancing, weightlifting, or playing a sport, having fun will make it more likely that you'll stick with it.
- Mix it up. Avoid monotony by incorporating variety into your routine. Trying new exercises, classes, or workout formats can keep things interesting and prevent boredom.

- Get an accountability partner. Partnering with a friend or joining group classes can provide accountability and motivation. Knowing someone is expecting you can make it harder to skip a workout.
- Reward yourself. Celebrate your achievements, no matter how small. Treat yourself to a healthy snack, a relaxing bath, or something you enjoy when you reach a fitness milestone.
- Track your progress. Keep a workout log or use fitness apps to track your progress. Seeing improvements over time can be motivating and reinforce your commitment.
- Establish a pre-workout routine. Develop a pre-workout routine that signals to your brain that it's time to exercise. This could include stretching, listening to energizing music, or having a quick, healthy snack.
- Set short term and long term goals. In addition to long term goals, set short term goals that you can achieve within a few weeks. These smaller victories can help maintain motivation.
- Be flexible. Life is unpredictable and there will be days when your original workout plan isn't feasible. Be flexible and willing to adapt your routine without feeling guilty.
- Positive self talk. Cultivate a positive mindset. Instead of focusing on what you can't do, celebrate what you can. Replace negative thoughts with affirmations that reinforce your commitment.
- Incorporate rest days. Rest is an essential component of any fitness routine. Give your body time to recover to prevent burnout and reduce the risk of injury.
- Visual reminders. Use visual cues to remind yourself of your fitness goals. This could be a vision board, post-it notes, or setting your workout gear in a visible location.
- Reassess and adjust. Periodically reassess your goals and adjust your workout routine accordingly. As your fitness level improves, you may need to increase intensity or try new challenges.

6

Conclusion

Remember that building a habit takes time, and setbacks are normal. Be patient with yourself and stay focused on the positive changes you're making for your health and well-being. It's also important to remember to start all workouts with a warm up and finish with a cool down like stretching to prevent injury and enhance flexibility. Adjust your intensity to each workout based on your fitness level and fitness goals. Feel free to mix and match exercises to keep your workouts diverse and enjoyable.

Good Luck on your fitness journey. I hope you've found this book to be beneficial and informative and that it helps you on your fitness quest.